EPSOM SALT

HOLISTIC RECIPES FOR BEAUTIFUL SKIN, PAIN RELIEF AND RELAXATION

BY SMART READS

1

Free Audiobook

As a thank you for being a Smart Reader you can choose 2 FREE audiobooks from audible.com. Simply sign up for free by visiting www.audibletrial.com/Travis to get your books.

Visit:
www.smartreads.co/freebooks
to receive Smart Reads books for FREE

Check us out on Instagram:
www.instagram.com/smart_readers
@smart_readers

ABOUT SMARTREADS

Choose Smart Reads and get smart every time. Smart Reads sorts through all the best content and condenses the most helpful information into easily digestible chunks.

We design our books to be short, easy to read and highly informative. Leaving you with maximum understanding in the least amount of time.

Smart Reads aims to accelerate the spread of quality information so we've taken the copyright off everything we publish and donate our material directly to the public domain. You can read our uncopyright below.

We believe in paying it forward and donate 5% of our net sales to Pencils of Promise to build schools, train teachers and support child education.

To limit our footprint and restore forests around the globe we are planting a tree for every 10 hardcover books we sell.

Thanks for choosing Smart Reads and helping us help the planet.

Sincerely,

Travis & the Smart Reads Team

TABLE OF CONTENTS

INTRODUCTION

Epsom salt, also known as magnesium sulfate, is a pure, time-tested compound, which has been used in numerous ways for hundreds of years. The salts, as they are sometimes called, are not actually salts but a naturally occurring mineral compound of magnesium and sulfate. The salts are named after the springs in Surrey England where these natural minerals were discovered in the water. They are a must-have natural remedy for any household. They can be used topically, or ingested, and have various uses.

More and more people are turning to natural remedies containing natural ingredients and no toxic chemicals. Rather than exposing yourself and your family to harsh chemicals, which can be found in a lot of modern medications, perhaps you can learn about more natural alternatives and the benefits they offer. Since natural remedies come from natural sources, like herbs, clean food, and essential oils, they are so much better and healthier for your body than chemically manufactured remedies made from factories.

This is where Epsom salts comes in. They are so versatile and a great option to explore. There is so much you can do with them, not only are they great for your physical body, but they can also enhance your home and even your garden. They can be used to assist in weight loss, flush out toxins from the body, ease migraines and headaches, promote relaxation, clean your house and also help your garden plants grow healthy. Keep a bag in the house at all times and you'll soon see what a difference these salts make.

This book is intended to guide you through the numerous uses for Epsom salts. It is also intended to advise you on exactly what to do with them and how to use them so that you gain maximum benefit. Once you realize how useful these salts are, you will make sure to always keep some around the house for anything you may need.

CHAPTER 1: EPSOM SALT BASICS

Using Epsom salts on your body is one of the best things you can do. They provide enormous benefits, from the relief of aches and pains, to helping with weight loss. Make sure you keep some around the house to help out when you need them. Some of you may remember Epsom salts hiding in your grandmother's medicine cabinet or at school a long time ago. Despite the length of time, Epsom salts is still a very popular solution for so many of today's most common ailments. There's a good reason they've been around for so long.

In the water where Epsom salts were found, is a mineral known as magnesium sulfate. As mentioned above, the name Epsom salts come from the English area where the salts were discovered and originally distilled from the water. You can buy these salts in supermarkets, health food stores, or pharmacies so they are easily available to everyone. The best part is, they don't cost much and are so versatile. Epsom salts have so many uses, the most common are for healing - relief of pain, healing sores or cuts, and even for improving the quality of skin and making grooming tasks easier.

Of course, the most popular way the salts have been used is in baths. When you draw a bath, only about a handful of salts are needed and can be thrown into the warm water. You'll soon feel the benefits it has to offer. It can make you feel a lot better and help melt away any stress, restoring a sense of calm, relieving sore or tense muscles, and getting your nervous system to unwind.

Another very important use for the salts is cleansing. Considering their constitution, their coarseness works well to exfoliate when they are added to warm water. They can also be used as a homemade facial mask that can help take away excess oil on the skin. If you're having a bad hair day or don't have not enough time to wash your hair, adding some Epsom salts can clean out the follicles making it easier to groom/comb your hair.

Epsom salts are also great for healing sprains and bruises. You can run a bath with Epsom salts, enough to cover the affected area. This will help to minimize any soreness, reduce swelling, and provide relief for areas that are hurt. Just ensure to keep the hurt parts of your body immersed in the water for around 20 minutes or longer if possible. It will help bring relief and also creates a relaxing feeling.

The salts can also ease migraines, reduce inflammation, assist with muscle and nerve function, regulate enzymes, flush out toxins, and much more. This is due to the very important role that magnesium plays in the human body.

Epsom Salt Usage

Epsom salts aren't anything new, they've been around and been used for hundreds of years, and have a proven record of making people feel better. Actually, you've probably already used Epsom salts at some point but haven't realized its full capacity as a helpful everyday compound.

Some of you may remember being at your grandparents' houses playing your little hearts out and falling over, getting bruised, or cutting your knees, for example. Perhaps you've had a really bad cold and flu symptoms and your muscles felt sore too. Do you remember taking a bath and it helped you relieve some cold and flu symptoms, or sore muscles? Did you feel soothed and more relaxed? Did it also help you sleep better at night?

If you remember anything like this from your childhood years, it is highly likely your grandparents or parents had put you in a bath and thrown in some Epsom salts.

The amazing thing about the Epsom salts is that they are not only beneficial and effective, but also very gentle. It does not matter what you are dealing with – cuts and bruises, colds and flus, removing splinters, relieving sore muscles etc.

Speaking of sore muscles, athletes often use Epsom salts for their sore muscles. Everyone, young or old, athlete or non-athlete can use them. Anyone can use these as a remedy for a myriad of ailments without having to worry about any side effects. Think about what other remedies or medication you can use that will provide all of these things.

There are so many great reasons for using Epsom salts in your everyday life. Some of them include:

1. Effective— Epsom salts are effective and provide benefits for anyone that uses them. They can make you feel better and help remedy the most common ailments. Within just minutes of usage, they can deliver great results compared to other medications that may or may not work. Sometimes, certain medications will take a few days to kick in and start working. Once you give Epsom salts a try you will love how fast it works and that side effects are almost nonexistent.

2. Inexpensive—Epsom salts are affordable, inexpensive items you can purchase to assist you with improving your body and your health. They cost only $3 or $4 for a bag but they can make a real difference to your general health. It is a fact that most medications will put quite a large dent in people's wallets every month and that every remedy must be paid for separately. For just a few dollars, you could get a fabulous remedy for only a fraction of the cost.

3. Versatile — Epsom salts can be used in so many different ways. Instead of buying a lot of different products that will do the same types of things, you could opt to spend your money on some Epsom salts and achieve the same result.

4. Safe—Because they are all-natural, Epsom salts are safe to use. They are great to use when you're feeling ill, sore, or just in a blue mood. So many medications aren't safe for use on children, or they have side effects, Epsom salts can help cure various issues, including that of your child's, without worry of side effects happening.

5. Purely Natural—This is one of the best things about Epsom salts – they're natural and contain no toxic or unnatural chemicals in them. This makes them the right choice for using on the body.

Epsom Salt Benefits

In many cases, people have only one or a few preferred uses for Epsom salts. It could be their usual choice when they feel they need something to help them relax after a long day, or perhaps they like to use them for taking care of bruises or other ailments that need a bit of extra care. Unfortunately, most people aren't aware of the many other ways that Epsom salts can be of use to them. Below are other ways Epsom salts can be used:

1. Relaxing—There's nothing better than finding some way to completely relax after a long and busy day or when in recovery after an illness. Adding two or three cups of Epsom salts into a warm bath then soaking in it for 20 minutes or more can help to refresh the mind, relax the body, and to help you to feel better.

2. Foot Scrubs—For some people, their feet are a source of pain or embarrassment, or both. Are yours beginning to look rough? Have you recently been working out and feel your feet need a bit of tender care? Epsom salts can be used to make a great foot scrub. This will eliminate dead skin cells, leaving your feet really soft. If you are not a fan of foot scrubs, you could add about one cup of salts to some hot/warm water and then soak your feet for around twenty minutes. This will relax you and also help with the healing of any cuts or bruises.

3. Removing splinters—To get this done, soak the affected area in some water with the Epsom salts in it. You should be able to remove the splinter more easily.

4. Relieve aches and pains —When you have a cold or perhaps you worked particularly hard on any given day and you feel your body is struggling, it might be the time to consider bringing out your Epsom salts. Draw a bath and throw in two cups of salts. Get in and soak for a minimum of 20 minutes. This will allow the magnesium to penetrate through your skin and begin relieving muscles and emotional stress.

5. Improving hair—A good way to give your hair more volume is by spraying some salt into it. This will not only add more volume but also improve the texture. Place Epsom salts into an atomizer with filtered water and spray it over your hair. You could also place Epsom salts directly into a hair conditioner bottle (equal parts conditioner and salts). When you apply it, leave it on your hair for about twenty minutes. This will add thickness and volume to thinning hair.

6. Headache relief—For people who suffer migraines or chronic headaches, Epsom salts can be a very simple solution. They are great in helping relieve headaches. If they are used in a bath they will bring even more health benefits.

7. Laxative—Epsom salts can also be used to help bowel movements whenever you are suffering from irregularity. They serve as gentle laxatives. All you have to do is dissolve one teaspoon into a bit of water, stir and drink.

8. Smoother skin—In order to get your skin feeling smooth you must exfoliate. This will expel any dead skin cells. Mix ¼ cup olive oil and ½ cup Epsom salts. Scrub this on your skin. It will help make your skin softer, more beautiful and healthier.

9. Minor sunburn—As summer hits, it's important to avoid sunburn especially since the sun's rays can be very powerful. To achieve relief from sunburn, take ½ cup of water and add a little Epsom salt into it. If you allow it to cool a little as well, it will provide some more relief. You can spray it onto the skin if it's too sensitive to touch.

10. Itchy skin or bug bites—Summer is not only notorious for sunburn but also bugs and bug bites. If you place a little Epsom salts into ½ cup of water then let it cool down, it can work well to relieve the itching. This can be used for simply itchy skin with no bug bites. You can use a wet compress or spray it into the affected areas.

11. Better sleep—Some parents have figured out that adding the salts to their kids' bathwater helps their children relax a little more and also fall asleep easier and deeper.

12. Removing toxins—Epsom salts are excellent in removing toxins from the body. With Epsom salts a lot of toxins can be eliminated and this will help you lose some weight easier as well as remain healthier.

13. Making insulin more effective—Proper magnesium and sulfate levels help increase the effectiveness of insulin inside the body. They can also lower the risk of diabetes.

14. Improving heart health—A lot of people concerned with their hearts use Epsom salts. The salts have the ability to improve circulation and help avoid hardening arteries or blood clots, which are two issues that need addressing for those concerned about health problems like heart failure.

15. Garden improvements—Adding only 1 tablespoon of Epsom salts to garden soil will help boost vegetable growth.

16. Watering house plants—If the plants in your house are looking a little droopy and perhaps need a bit of help, just add a few tablespoons of Epsom salts to the watering can.

17. Removing slugs—If slugs have become an issue for you in your garden or patio sprinkle a little Epsom salt around the problem areas. Epsom salt will not bother you, however, it will deter slugs.

18. Cleaning grout—If your bathroom is beginning to look a bit grimy and you can't seem to get all the tiles clean then add dish soap and Epsom salts in equal parts then scrub the affected areas. Rinse well afterwards to ensure there are no streaks.

Epsom salts are such a versatile product to buy and use. They can help in so many ways and is gentle enough for anybody to use. For those of you who might be suffering from any problems listed above, seriously consider getting yourself Epsom salts and begin using them.

CHAPTER 2: WEIGHT LOSS USING EPSOM SALTS

One of the most popular uses for Epsom salts is, you guessed it, weight loss. People are almost always trying to lose excess weight, whether it is only a few pounds or a lot more. For some people it is only a matter of a small number of "vanity pounds." For others, it may be a matter of prioritizing their health after a scare, a doctor's advice, or because they generally want to make some changes in their lifestyle.

Whatever it is for you, there are a few options available that will help you lose some weight. Just be careful which ones you choose as some of them are not healthy. A lot of fad diets don't work and can sometimes be dangerous. A better option would be to change some of the food items you eat, choose whole foods more often instead of processed food, and start using your Epsom salts more.

For many years now, Epsom salts have been promoted as one solution to help people lose weight. There are ways you can incorporate Epsom salts into your life and they can help with weight loss. However, keep in mind that you still need to pair it with exercise and a better diet. By themselves alone, Epsom salts won't make you lose weight. They can be used as part of a process that can help make weight loss a little easier.

Epsom Baths for Weight Loss

One way you might want to utilize Epsom salts for weight loss is to add them to a warm bath. As mentioned, adding the salts to a bath will help with relaxation after a long day or intense workout, but can also be helpful in weight loss. Of course, as with anything, this will not magically occur overnight, nor will it occur solely because of the salts. However, Epsom salts can and are a helpful tool to use when trying to lose some weight. Relaxing your mind and body will also have some added effects for weight loss. A stressed person naturally craves carbs, and lots of them. If you are more relaxed your body will not necessarily need high carb food. This is one way it can help you reduce your calorie and carbohydrate intake during the day.

Epsom baths will also help eliminate toxins that have built up in the body. Let's face it, today we are surrounded with unnatural chemicals, artificially processed foods and other goods, and it's not unusual for people to start holding toxins in the body. When toxins are eliminated there is more potential for losing weight as well as even more potential to absorb great nutrients, and remain healthier.

Another benefit of having a salt bath is it will relax tired muscles. After working out it will be easier to work out again the next day and see even more results. Epsom salts added to your bath will give your muscles a much-needed break as well as bring a rejuvenating touch to your spirit. This will help you get back into life, your workouts, your job etc. again the next day.

Even though Epsom salts are not directly responsible for weight loss, they certainly are involved in an indirect manner by eliminating toxins from your body and helping you relax a bit more. Epsom salts will also help reinvigorate your muscles so you're ready to face another day.

Epsom Salt Drinks for Weight Loss
In some cases, people choose to drink Epsom salts as a way of losing weight. In such cases, it is necessary to mention that Epsom salts themselves are not a type of magical pill for weight loss. You can indeed drink the salts, however you must be careful. Epsom salts will work as laxatives within the body so take care when drinking them. The salts and the water in the body will bind together and make your stool softer and therefore easier to pass.

Just like laxatives in general, it's possible for people to lose pounds after using them. However, a word of caution: drinking Epsom salts (especially if you overdo it) could end up giving you a lot of other issues such as nausea, vomiting, and diarrhea, and become dehydrated instead. In this case, you would not actually be losing fat but water weight, so there won't be any weight loss benefits in this. **For this reason, Epsom salts are not really recommended for drinking. Should you decide to do so, please proceed with care.**

Epsom Salt Recipes
Weight loss using Epsom salts has been encouraged since the early 1900's. The recipes below are intended to help relieve issues you might have with losing weight. They are quite simple to follow and anyone can do them.

Weight Loss Salt Bath
Ingredients:
1 tub of hot water
2 cups Epsom Salts

Directions:
1. For weight loss using an Epsom salt bath, ensure the bath is filled with some hot water to the level you prefer.

2. Add two full cups of the Epsom salts then swirl the water around to make sure it all gets mixed in well.
3. Get yourself into your bath tub and enjoy the feeling of warm water over your body for twenty minutes at least and allow the Epsom salts do their work, helping you reduce stress levels.
4. Rinse yourself off completely before drying off.

Epsom Salt Drinks

Ingredients:
1 cup water (lemon juice is ok too if you prefer)
1 tablespoon Epsom salts

Directions:
1. For a weight loss drink, you place one tablespoon Epsom salts to one cup of lemon juice or water, whatever you prefer.
2. Drink it only once daily and even then just for 2 or 3 days. This will ensure you avoid any problems.

CHAPTER 3: USING EPSOM SALTS FOR RELAXATION AND PAIN RELEIF

These salts are well-known for their pain reducing abilities and for the way they can allow the body to relax faster. In today's world everyone is so busy, always rushing around doing this and doing that. We have things to get done for school, for work, for the family etc. Often, our schedules can give us a lot of stress even without us knowing it. When you feel stressed it makes it really difficult to relax.

To make matters worse, so many people are also living with physical pain of some kind every day. For some it's bad headaches, for others it's other aches and pains. Back pain is a major stressor and is experienced by millions of people. For others, their jobs are strenuous and they are on their feet all day or lugging heavy things around. Perhaps people are dealing with inflammation as well which makes life so much more difficult.

There are, in fact, a lot of different types of pain experienced by individuals. It may be mild or it may be severe, but it will still take a toll on the body nonetheless. It also makes life difficult to enjoy. A lot of people take medication to manage the pain and often this medication will come with side effects.

Finding a better, more natural approach to deal with pain is something many people prefer.

For so many years, people have used Epsom salts to treat pain and inflammation and to help with relaxation. Epsom salts has been and continues to be a popular treatment for the relief of sore muscles and also other types of aches and pains. While people may think that this is only folklore and Epsom salts don't really work as promised, there have been several studies clearly showing how Epsom salts are an effective healing remedy for the treatment of many conditions associated with pain in the body. In addition, this simple yet effective treatment is available over the counter and not expensive at all.

How Epsom Salts Assist with the Relief of Pain
Muscle aches and pains can originate from different sources. At times it can be the result of overworking for the day and at other times, it can come from a particular medical condition like fibromyalgia or rheumatoid arthritis.

A lot of bodily aches and pains, whether they are because of a medical condition or not, can be relieved by using Epsom salts.

Epsom salts work to relieve such pains, including muscle pain, through its key ingredient, magnesium. Magnesium is an essential mineral for the body, helping it to function properly. The big difference with magnesium is that it can be absorbed quickly through the skin, so if you are sitting in a hot bath, this mineral will easily make its way into your system.

The important uses magnesium can provide for the body are numerous. They're especially good at relaxing the skeletal muscles because they can easily flush out lactic acid which can make muscles sore especially during and after physical exertion like exercise, hard physical work, or during times of inflammation. Lactic acid builds up during these periods but the magnesium in Epsom salts will help to flush this out and allow other vitamins and minerals to be absorbed by the body quicker as well. To add to this, magnesium helps regulate not only muscle function, but also nerve function.

The easiest and, let's face it, probably the most enjoyable way to relieve and soothe muscles is by getting into a nice, warm bath with Epsom salts. A full tub (or lower level if you prefer) with 1 or 2 cups of the salts will be enough to relieve most aches people experience. A footbath is another great idea and is fantastic for sore, tired feet at the end of the day. If there are other body parts that need pain relief you can make a small bath, perhaps even using a bucket with some warm water and Epsom salts. Place the affected part into the water and soak for about 20 minutes.

Again, it will provide you with, not only sore muscle relief, but the ability to properly relax. If you are tired and sore it is a lot harder to relax, and having pain makes people tense up even more. Sometimes, people worry about the pain they are experiencing and whether it will ever go away. This gives them even more stress! Perhaps you could also add lavender essential oil or an oil of your choosing to the Epsom salt bath. Just make sure the essential oils you use are A-grade, pure oils.

Recipes
Epsom salts are useful in dealing with pain relief as well as assisting in the relaxation process. The recipes below will make things easier for you and will also ensure you get all the pain relief and relaxation your body needs and deserves.

Relaxing the Body (and by extension, the mind)

Ingredients:
½ cup Epsom salts

2 teaspoons baking soda
10 drops of lavender oil

Directions:
1. In an appropriate sized bowl, combine all the ingredients above until they are combined well.
2. Go to the bath, turn on taps and arrange the temperature that you feel comfortable with. Pour the ingredients inside the bowel into the bath and mix the water around well.
3. Step into your bath, sit back and soak your body for a minimum of twenty minutes. This will give the Epsom salts enough time to really do a good job.
4. Don't use any soap on the body after the soak as it will take off the above recipe therefore taking away its effectiveness.

Re-energizing

Ingredients:
½ cup of Epsom salts
2 tsp. of baking soda
10 drops of eucalyptus essential oil
2 drops of lemon essential oil

Directions:
1. Place all the above ingredients into a bowl and make sure they are combined well.

2. Now pour the mixture into a bath that's already prepared with hot water. Give it one or two minutes until it mixes in well.

3. Get yourself into the tub and just enjoy all the feelings of relaxation and the scents for at least 20 minutes.

4. Dry yourself when done.

5. Enjoy the feeling of renewal and heightened energy.

Fabulous Foot Soaks

Ingredients:
1 pan of warm water
½ cup of Epsom Salts

Directions:
1. On the stovetop warm some water for only 2 or 3 minutes. Then add the Epsom salt mixture and stir to combine well.

2. Put your feet in the water. Let them soak. When the warm water isn't warm any more take them out.

3. Sometimes you might like more than the few minutes of soaking so you can reheat this water then start again. Once you feel complete rinse off your feet and dry them.

4. The recipe above is great for athlete's foot, nail fungi, and any type of sore feet.

Inflammation and Gout

Ingredients:
5 drops of orange essential oil
1 bucket of hot water
3 tsp. of Epsom Salts

Directions:
1. Pour hot water into your container until it's full. Try to make it hot to the extent you can handle. Add the salts and orange essential oil. You can add any essential oil of your choosing but orange is great for its uplifting and cleansing qualities.
2. Put your feet (or foot) into the container with water and allow them to soak around 30 minutes or so.

Uplifting Moods

Ingredients:
1 tub warm water
1 cup Epsom Salts
6 drops of sandalwood essential oil

Directions:
1. Fill your tub with nice, warm water to a level you prefer.

2. While this is occurring, combine Epsom salts and sandalwood essential oils and pour them into the bath. Swirl the water.
3. Get yourself into the warm bath and soak in its warmness allowing all the scents to uplift your mood and help you feel better.
4. Dry yourself off and get on with your day.

Immunity Boost

Ingredients:
1 cup Epsom salts
1 cup baking soda
7 ½ cups ginger
1 cup vinegar (apple cider)
1 cup sea salt

Directions:

1. Begin filling the tub with water. Make it as hot as you can handle.
2. While tub is being filled, in a bowl combine the sea and Epsom salts, vinegar, and baking soda.
3. Measure one cup of the mixture and add it to the tub. Now also add one cup of the apple cider vinegar. Swirl it all around.

4. Get yourself into the bathtub and allow yourself to soak for around 40 minutes. This will help your immune system.

CHAPTER 4: BEAUTY AND RADIANT SKIN

A beauty regimen and a good skin care routine is sought after these days. People, especially women, will do lots of research on this topic and often shell out a lot of money for products that claim to do a myriad of things. Some people worry what their skin looks like, if they have acne and how to clear it, what their hair looks like, if they have soft lips or cracked lips etc. The following recipes are great and very easy to organize in order to have fabulous skin and natural beauty without having to shell so much money.

RECIPES

Hair Volume

Ingredients:
1 tablespoon conditioner of your choice
1 tablespoon of Epsom Salts

Directions:
1. For hair that is a little drab and dull and you would like to give it some volume and a lift just combine the above ingredients together.
2. It's a good idea to warm the mixture a bit before you work it through your hair. Once applied to the hair evenly, leave it in for around 15 minutes or so.

3. Rinse off mixture from the hair and just enjoy your new hair volume.

For Acne

Ingredients:
½ cup hot water
4 drops of iodine
1 tsp. of Epsom salts

Directions:
1. A good way to clean the face and remove excess oil is through exfoliation. This will also help with acne.
2. The exfoliating mixture will consist of water, Epsom salts and iodine. Stir the ingredients together and make sure they have all been dissolved. Allow the mixture to set. This may take a couple of minutes.
3. Then massage the mixture onto your skin and let it dry completely before washing it off your face.

Oily Hair Solution

Ingredients:
1 cup Epsom salts, and
1 cup lemon juice

Directions:

1. In a pot of water, combine lemon juice, Epsom salts and stir well. Place the lid on top and let it set for about 24 hours, after which time it should be ready to use.
2. Once it's ready, pour this mixture all over your hair and keep it on the hair for 20 minutes to let it do its work.
3. Once the 20 minutes is up, wash and condition your hair as per usual.

Lip Balm

Ingredients:
2 tbsp. of Epsom salts
1 tsp. of petroleum jelly

Directions:
1. Place the salts and petroleum jelly together.
2. Massage the mixture gently onto your lips. This will take away the dead skin cells and leave your lips feeling soft.
3. Once this is done, wipe it off your lips. Enjoy the softness.

Bath Bombs

Ingredients:
1 tsp. of vanilla extract

½ cup Epsom salt
1 cup baking soda
½ cup citric acid
2 tsp. of olive oil
2 tsp. of witch hazel

Directions:
1. For the bath bomb recipe, combine baking soda, salt, and citric acid together then mix until they are all combined well. In a separate bowl, combine olive oil, vanilla and witch hazel.
2. Once everything is well mixed you can add these liquid ingredients together with the dry ingredients. Mix them all using your hands. This is the best way to do it.
3. Press mixture into silicon molds then press firmly. Set these aside until they become hard. You will be able to store them for about 2 weeks in a container.

CHAPTER 5: EPSOM SALTS AND YOUR GARDEN

Gardening is an enjoyable pastime and one that many people enjoy. Getting outside in the sunshine and fresh air is good for you. Growing your own food is also great for your health. So many vegetables can be grown in your own backyard or even a makeshift indoor garden. You don't need a huge amount of space to grow things in your garden and depending what you choose to grow, you don't even need to put in too much time either. Epsom salts may not be the first thing people think about when gardening but they can actually help your garden grow lusher.

Gardening with Epsom Salts

Some of you may feel your gardens are not growing as lush as you want them too, or perhaps your plants or veggies look a little withered. Epsom salts are great for gardens and using the salts is a very economic and versatile way of caring for it.

Many people wonder how Epsom salts can help their gardens. The answer is easy: magnesium and sulfate. These are both found inside salts and will also do wonders for your garden. Epsom salts serve as better fertilizers because they don't build up in the soil. They're also easy and safe to use.

First, let's discuss magnesium. It is a good mineral to put into your garden when the seeds you've planted are just beginning to grow. It helps the seeds germinate and strengthens the plants' cell walls, which in turn allows for more nutrients to enter. In addition, magnesium is important for plants since it helps them with photosynthesis. If plants don't have enough magnesium, their seeds will struggle to absorb enough phosphorus and nitrogen, even if they are plentiful in the soil. Adding just a small amount of Epsom salt to your garden will increase your crops and you'll get more for all your gardening efforts.

Second, there's sulfate. It is the mineral form of sulfur and it's found in abundance in nature. It is also important to plant life. Proper sulfate levels help plants produce chlorophyll and thus allows the plant to live longer. Sulfate inside soil will help nutrients already present to be more useful to the plant. When sulfate is in the soil, it mixes with phosphorus, potassium, and nitrogen; together they help plants grow bigger and stronger. Sulfate and magnesium work well together to provide gardens with nourishment, no matter what type of garden you have or where it's located.

Of course, it's possible to have a lovely garden without using Epsom salts, however, the salts will make a very noticeable difference to how your garden grows. For first time gardeners, or those who are having trouble getting their gardens to thrive, Epsom salts is the main ingredient to have.

Epsom Salt in Your Garden
For those with limited space or those who prefer a smaller garden, potted plants are a great solution. With potted plants, you have more options available on where you grow your plants, including indoors if you would like to. Sometimes, growing plants inside might be a bit of a challenge because you have to ensure they are in a place that gets enough sunlight. Sometimes there are problems with the air quality and sometimes it's with the quality of the soil. Epsom salts can be a big help for your flowers and your plants' health.

Adding some Epsom salts to potted plants will only take a couple of minutes. Add 2 tablespoons of salt for every gallon. Use this mixture one time each month instead of plain watering on that day. Your potted plants will benefit from it.

Using Epsom salts from the very beginning of a plant's life is also a good idea. You could take garden soil you'd like to grow your plants in and add Epsom salts to it. The soil can either be from ground that has been fertilized already, or perhaps store bought potting soil. It doesn't matter which one you choose you can still add Epsom salts. One cup of salt will work for one hundred square feet. Work the salt into your soil just before you put in the plants or seeds. This will help plants to grow strong and the seeds to germinate.

Use salts whenever you feel your garden is not growing as well as you'd like it to or your plants aren't as strong. Place about 2 tablespoons of Epsom salts for every gallon of water and water your plants with this, one or two times a month. You will see a difference in the lushness and beauty of your garden.

If you have a vegetable garden, they could also benefit enormously if you use Epsom salts. Of course, all plants will love the salt but there are a huge number of vegetables that will be able to use them to grow even better than usual. These include tomatoes and peppers because they often have insufficient magnesium. When these types of vegetables lack proper magnesium levels, they will have lower yields and leaves that turn yellow. Epsom salts can help solve this problem and allow the yield to be fuller. The magnesium will also not build up within the soil the way other chemicals sometimes do.

Other gardening areas that will reap the benefit if you use Epsom salt include the lawn area, which will become lusher and greener, flower gardens, and also any trees that you might have. Epsom salts are very versatile. They can have uses for almost everything that grows in a backyard. The best part is that you can't really go wrong when using them. In fact, you'll be amazed at how well they will work.

Gardening Recipes
At any point you decide it's time to start adding Epsom salts to your garden for an increased yield, try some of the recipes below.

For Greener Foliage

Ingredients:
½ gallon of water
1 Tbsp. of Epsom salts

Directions:
1. Firstly, add some Epsom salts to the water. The rule is that for every 12 inches of garden height you will pour this particular amount onto the soil.
2. You can do this instead of regular watering once a month. You can do this for your grass, shrubs,

vegetable garden, and your trees. Then sit back and enjoy the results.

Leaf Curling Antidote

Ingredients:
1 gallon of water
2 Tbsp. of Epsom salts

Directions:
1. Should you notice that the leaves on your plants are curling, it might be due to magnesium deficiency in your garden.
2. Add 2 tablespoons Epsom salts to 1 gallon water and then apply it directly to the plant leaves, and to your soil as well.
3. You'll soon notice the nutrients balancing themselves out and their leaves will start looking much better.

Larger Productions

Ingredients:
1 tsp. of Epsom salts
1 gallon of water
Directions:

1. We all want to get a lot of produce from our plants during summer in particular, and this is a recipe that can make this happen.
2. Firstly, fill the sprayer with water and add only 1 teaspoon of the Epsom salts. Spray this recipe onto your plants preferably every week. This will help to create great produce.

CHAPTER 6: CLEANING YOUR HOME USING EPSOM SALT

For some of you, keeping a clean home might seem like something you can only dream about. Of course, we all want our homes to look good and not be embarrassing when visitors come over. However, we all have so many other obligations and things we must take care of that cleaning might seem like a lower priority.

Epsom salts are great for helping keep your home clean. Some of you may need to disinfect certain areas of your home so as to keep flu and other viruses away. Perhaps you want to clean grout in your bathroom or other hard-to-reach parts of your home. Epsom salts can help you with this.

For the most part, household cleaners can keep the house clean but are usually full of toxic chemicals that are harmful to your health, and in particular to the health of young children. Even though these cleaning products might do a good job at cleaning, they're not usually safe to use or be around.

It is for this reason that many people are now turning to alternative cleaning materials for their homes and even offices. Epsom salts can provide this as they are all-natural and feature great cleansing abilities so they are safe to have around the home. In addition, they cost less than store-bought household cleaners. Seriously consider using Epsom salts for cleaning in your home.

Recipes

So many areas of homes need regular cleaning, especially rooms like the kitchen where food is prepared. Toxic cleaners leave streaks and chemicals that can come into contact with your food. Below are some recipes using the all-natural Epsom salts to keep your home clean and looking amazing.

Grout Cleaning

Ingredients:
1 cup dish detergent
1 cup Epsom salts

Directions:
1. In a bowl, mix the detergent and Epsom salts. Apply the mixture to any dirty or stained surface inside the bathroom, kitchen, or even outside.
2. Allow this mixture to sit for a few minutes and soak.
3. Start scrubbing until the grime is gone.
4. Lastly, rinse off the mixture to achieve a great shine.
5. Store remainder of mixture for later use.

Cleaning your Washer

Ingredients:
1 qt. of clear vinegar
1 cup Epsom salts

Directions:
1. Fill your washing machine with hot water.
2. Once it's filled, pour the quart of vinegar as well as the salts.
3. Let the washing machine agitate the mixture for around 1 minute and stop the cycle. Allow the solution to sit and soak inside the washer for about an hour before you put it on rinse cycle to drain.

Car Battery Regeneration

Ingredients:
½ cup of water
1 oz. Epsom salts

Directions:
1. Heat some water and make it very warm.
2. Place the Epsom salts in the water and make a paste.
3. Place some of the paste on each battery cell and watch them regenerate.

Ink Stains Be Gone

Ingredients:
Milk
Epsom salts

Directions:
1. Use some Epsom salts and rub them into the affected fabric. How much you need will depend on the particular area.
2. Then soak that fabric in some of the milk, which will help to get rid of the stain. It is better if you can keep the fabric in the milk overnight.
3. Finally, wash fabric as usual and any ink stains should disappear completely.

Removal of Mildew

Ingredients:
1 tsp. of Epsom salts
2 tsp. of lemon juice

Direction:
1. Mix both the ingredients above until they form a paste. If you are dealing with a larger area just double or even tripe the amount.

2. Put this paste on areas that have mildew and allow it to set. This will probably take only a few minutes. Scrub clean.

Wine Stain Removal

Ingredients:
Water
1 Tbsp. of Epsom salts

Directions:
1. Wine stain on a favorite shirt? Lay it flat out and then sprinkle enough Epsom salts to cover the affected area.
2. Allow the fabric to soak up the liquid.
3. Soak the affected fabric for around one hour in cold water then wash it as usual.
4. The stain will have disappeared.

Toilet Cleaning

Ingredients:
2 Tbsp. Epsom salts
1 cup baking soda
1/3 cup citric acid
30 drops of lemon essential oil
20 drops of orange essential oil

Directions:
1. In a bowl, stir the Epsom salts, baking soda, and citric acid. Add only a spritz of some water to help dampen the mixture. Mix well with your hands.
2. Once combined, stir the essential oils in and continue mixing so it will all come together.
3. Now spoon the mixture onto a baking sheet that is lined with parchment paper. Allow this to set - at least a 24 hour period to let it harden.
4. Then store this in a dry, cool place. When it's ready for you to use, place one into the toilet water and let it fizz. Scrub clean and enjoy the shininess!

Hand Wash Mixture

Ingredients:
2 Tbsp. of Epsom salts
1 cup baby oil
3 drops of jasmine essential oil
3 drops of vanilla essential oil

Directions:
1. Take a bowl and combine Epsom salts and baby oil. Stir the mixture until it is very well combined.
2. Now pour mixture into a hand wash plastic bottle and place it near your sink or basin. Use when needed to keep hands clean and soft.

Bug Spray

Ingredients:
2 Tbsp. of Epsom salts
16 oz. of warm water
5-6 drops of tea tree essential oil
5-6 drops of lemon essential oil
5-6 drops of citronella essential oil

Directions:
1. Get a large spray bottle and pour Epsom salts inside it. Fill the bottle with warm water but leave a little room at the top.
2. To dissolve the salts shake the bottle well. Add the 3 essential oils and shake as you add each one so that everything mixes together well.
3. Spray the mixture onto yourself or your plants. This will ensure bugs and other pests will stay away.

Kitchen Sink Cleaner

Ingredients:
4 cups of hot water
1 cup Epsom salts
10 drops lemon essential oil
10 drops eucalyptus essential oil

Directions:

1. Add the Epsom salts into the hot water and stir until the Epsom salts dissolve completely. Now add the lemon and eucalyptus essential oils.

2. After you've cleaned the sink, pour some of the mixture into the drain. Now run hot water down into it and this should erase any odors hiding in your sink. You might need one more shot at this if the mixture wasn't enough, but usually just one time is sufficient.

CHAPTER 7: EPSOM SALT MEDICINAL USES

People deal with a myriad of health conditions from one day to the next. It might be sore muscles, the flu, or a splinter. Of course, these are not serious health issues but they are issues nonetheless and they can still put a damper on anyone's day. They can also make it harder to get things done, whether it is around your home or in your workplace.

Often, when people experience common ailments such as those mentioned above, they might reach for one of their usual medications. While medication can be necessary at times and also effective at relieving some common ailments, it can also leave certain side effects and is usually more expensive to buy.

The good news is that Epsom salts can assist in relieving many common ailments as well. Even better news is that they don't have any side effects like most modern medications. Plus, they're also affordable.

Below are some recipes you can use for relieving common medical issues using Epsom salts.

RECIPES

Removing Splinters

Ingredients
8 oz. of hot water
1 tsp. of Epsom salt

Directions:
1. You will need to make a paste for this particular recipe in order to remove a splinter. Using a bowl, place the hot water and add the Epsom salts.
2. Now stir the mixture until the salts are completely dissolved and put this mixture into the fridge for about 20 minutes.
3. Once the time is over, take it out of your fridge and clean off any affected areas. Pat dry and then apply a layer of paste onto affected area(s).
4. Now cover it with a bandage and allow it to sit for half an hour. After the time is up, the splinter should come out easily.

Compress for Poison Ivy

Ingredients:
1 cup of cold water
2 Tbsp. of Epsom salts
1 drop of lavender essential oil
1 drop of tea tree essential oil

Directions:

1. In a bowl, combine Epsom salts and water together and then stir well so that the salts are completely dissolved.

2. Once the salts are dissolved, add the lavender and tea tree essential oils and mix again until fully combined.

3. Take a washcloth and soak it in the solution. When it's ready, place it on the affected body part.

4. Allow the washcloth to sit on the affected area until it is no longer cold. Repeat this treatment at any time or whenever relief is needed.

Postnatal Bath Bombs

Ingredients:

1 cup baking soda
½ cup Epsom salt
¼ teaspoon of plantain leaf
¼ teaspoon of dried lavender
¼ teaspoon of comfrey
¼ teaspoon of calendula
½ cup of citric acid
1 teaspoon of vanilla
½ tablespoon of olive oil
½ tablespoon of water

Directions:

1. When a woman has a baby there is often associated pain. There is also the need to relax. This recipe is perfect to add to your after baby routine.

2. First of all, take a large bowl and add the Epsom salts, baking soda, and citric acid together.

3. Using another bowl, whisk the olive oil, vanilla, and water together. Once they are combined, pour them into the other dry ingredients. Mix them all together with your hands and then add the herbs.

4. Once this is done, divide the mixture and place into silicone molds. Press the mixture in well and leave it in the molds for 24 hours (or more if you can) until the mixture hardens.

5. Remove them from the mold and store them until they are ready to use. When you need one just throw it into your hot bath. Allow it to fizz and then step into the bath and enjoy.

Tension Headache

Ingredients:
1 tub of hot water
2 cups Epsom salts
5 drops of Roman chamomile essential oil and
5 drops of rosemary oil

Directions:

1. Draw a bath with the water temperature you prefer. As the water is running, pour in the Epsom salts.
2. Add in the essential oils a few drops at a time. Make sure you swirl around the water so the oils spread all along and also to make sure the salts are properly dissolved.
3. When the Epsom salts have dissolved, turn off water and get into the tub. Allow the warm water to soothe you as you soak in it for at least half an hour.
4. When you are done pat yourself dry. You should be experiencing relief from the headaches and feeling more relaxed.

Bug Bite Relief

Ingredients:
1 cup warm water
2 tablespoons of Epsom salts
3 drops of lavender essential oil

Directions:
1. In a large enough bowl, place the Epsom salts in some water. Add the lavender essential oil and then continue stirring until all the salts dissolve.
2. Take a cotton ball and dip it into the mixture. Dab it directly onto affected area(s).
3. Allow the mixture to air dry. Just be careful not to scratch the affected area(s).

Body Detox

Ingredients:
½ cup Epsom salts
½ Tbsp. of water
5 drops of lemon oil
2 Tbsp. of coconut oil
1 tsp. of vanilla
1 cup baking soda
½ cup citric acid

Directions:
1. These detoxing bath bombs are great and easy to make. Stir citric acid together with the baking soda and Epsom salts.
2. In another bowl whisk the coconut oil, vanilla, and water together. Once all wet ingredients have been combined, just mix them together with the other dry ingredients. Do this with your hands.
3. Now add the lemon oil. If you need to add some more water to get the mixture sticking well then do so.
4. At this point you will divide this mixture and place it into silicone molds. Press it in very well. Allow the molds to set for at least one day so they have time to harden.

5. Once bath bombs have been prepared and are ready, remove them from their molds and use or store for about two weeks.
6. Just throw one into the tub when you need it and allow it to fizz.

Bee Stings

Ingredients:
1 cup cold water
2 Tbsp. of Epsom salts
1 drop peppermint essential oil
1 drop of lavender essential oil
1 drop of German chamomile essential oil

Directions:
1. Combine cold water and Epsom salts in a bowl. Stir until all the salts are completely dissolved before you add the peppermint and lavender essential oils.
2. Once they are all mixed together well, place a washcloth in this solution and soak it. Place it directly onto the affected area(s).
3. Keep it on the sting until it is no longer cold. Repeat the treatment as needed. This might be two or three times.

Insomnia and General Sleep Help

Ingredients:
Hot water
2 cups Epsom salts
5 drops of lavender essential oil
5 drops of Roman chamomile essential oil

Directions:
1. While you fill a bath and the water is running, pour in the Epsom salts.
2. Add the lavender and chamomile essential oils slowly, little drops at a time. This way they will be mixed in well. Swirl the bath water a little so the oils can spread out and the Epsom salts dissolve.
3. When everything has been dissolved and the bath is full, turn off the water. Get into the tub and relax, soaking for at least half an hour.
4. Dry yourself off and prepare to sleep well.

Clean Foot Solution

Ingredients:
½ cup Epsom salt
4 drops of eucalyptus essential oil
4 drops of orange essential oil
2 quarts of warm water

Directions:

1. Use a basin that is large enough to put your feet in and pour some warm water into it. Stir the ½ cup of Epsom salts and add the essential oils then swirl the water to make sure they are all mixed well.

2. Put this basin on the floor and put your feet into it. Soak them for around 20 minutes.

3. Once 20 minutes is over, remove your feet from the basin, then use the Epsom salt scrub to scrub your feet.

4. Rinse your feet off using warm water. Pat dry.

CONCLUSION

This book serves as a guide for you to learn about the many uses of Epsom salts and the reasons why you should consider buying some and using them in your life. Many people have heard of Epsom salts but perhaps haven't used them – until now.

Epsom salts are all natural, easy to use, not to mention, affordable. They can be used in so many different ways. Choosing to use natural and versatile products in your home is good for your health as well as your budget. Give Epsom salts a try right now.

THANKS FOR READING

We really hope you enjoyed this book. If you found this material helpful feel free to share it with friends. You can also help others find it by leaving a review where you purchased the book. Your feedback will help us continue to write books you love.

The Smart Reads library is growing by the day! Make sure and check out the other wonderful books in our catalog. We would love to hear which books are your favorite.

Visit:
www.smartreads.co/freebooks
to receive Smart Reads books for FREE

Check us out on Instagram:
www.instagram.com/smart_readers
@smart_readers

Don't forget your 2 FREE audiobooks.
Use this link www.audibletrial.com/Travis to claim
your 2 FREE Books.

SMART READS ORIGINS

Smart Reads was born out of the desire to find the best information fast without having to wade through the sheer volume of fluff available online. Smart Reads combs through massive amounts of knowledge compiles the best into quick to read books on a variety of subjects.

We consider ourselves Smart Readers, not dummies. We know reading is smart. We're self taught. We like to learn a TON about a WIDE variety of topics. We have developed a love for books and we find intelligence attractive.

We found that each new topic we tried to learn about started with the challenge of finding the pieces of the puzzle that mattered most. It becomes a treasure hunt rather than an education.

Smart Reads wants to find the best of the best information for you. To condense it into a package that you can consume in an hour or less. So you can read more books about more topics in less time.

OUR MISSION

Smart Reads aims to accelerate the availability of useful information and will publish a high quality book on every major topic on amazon.

Smart Reads hopes to remove barriers to sharing by taking the copyright off everything we publish and donating it to the public domain. We hope other publishers and authors will follow our example.

Our goal is to donate $1,000,000 or more by 2020 to build over 2,000 schools by giving 5% of our net profit to Pencils of Promise.

We want to restore forests around the globe by planting a tree for every 10 physical books we sell and hope to plant over 100,000 trees by 2020.

Doesn't it feel good knowing that by educating yourself you are helping the world be a better place? We think so too...

Thanks for helping us help the world. You Smart Reader you...

Travis and the Smart Reads Team

WHY I STARTED SMART READS

Every time I wanted to learn about something new I'd have to buy 20 books on the topic and spend way too long sorting through them and reading them all until I arrived at the big picture. Until I had enough perspectives to know who was just guessing, who was uninformed and who had stumbled upon something remarkable.

I wished someone else could just go in and figure that out for me and tell me what matters. That's how smart reads was born. I want smart reads to be a company that does all that research up front. Sorts through all the content that is available on each topic and pulls out the most up to date complete understanding, then have people smarter than me package the best wisdom in an easy to understand way in the least amount of words possible.

For example, I got a new puppy so I wanted to learn about dog training. I bought 14 different books about dog training and by the time I got through the first 5 and finally started getting the big picture on the best way to train my puppy she had grown up into a dog.

Yeah she's well behaved. She doesn't poop in the house. I can get her to sit and come when I call. But what if someone else went in and read all those books for me, found the underlying themes and picked out the best information that would give me the big picture and get me right to the point. And I'd only have to read one book instead of 15.

That would be amazing. I would save time. And maybe my dog would be rolling over, cleaning up after my kids and doing the dishes by now. That my friend, is the reason I started smart reads. Because I wanted a company I can trust to deliver me the best information in an easy to understand way that I can digest in under an hour. Because dog training is one of many subjects I want to master.

The quicker I can learn a wide variety of topics the sooner that information can begin playing a role in shaping my future. And none of us knows how long that future will be. So why not do everything we can to make the best of it and consume a ton of knowledge. And I figured all the better if I can also make a positive difference in the world.

That's why we're also building schools, planting trees and challenging ideas about copyright's place in today's world. Because as a company we have to be doing everything we can to support the ecosystem that gives us all these beautiful places to read our books. Thanks for reading.

Travis

Customers Who Bought This Book Also Bought

The Powerful Benefits of Myrrh: Effective Myrrh Recipes For Healthy & Beauty, Oil Pulling Therapy, Creativity, Aromatherapy and Improving The Mint

Beginner Gardening: Growing Vegetables and Ornamentals

Eating Clean: Detox, Reduce Weight, Fight Inflammation and Reset Your Body

Mint As Medicine: Discover The Powerful Healing Properties of Herb in Treating Headaches, Allergies, Asthma, Clarity and Peace of Mind

Natural Ways of Boosting Testosterone: How to Bulk Up and Put Your Sex Drive in Overdrive

Probiotic Dieting: The Miracle of Probiotics in Healing Your Gut, Trimming Belly Fat and Weight Loss